*Heal*

# Your Gut

## Change Your Life

### STEP BY STEP GUIDE TO THE GAPS DIET

### +50 RECIPES TO NOURISH & REPAIR

# Other Books by Andre Parker

Do you love bread but you have food intolerances?
Do you have a sensitive or even damaged digestive system?
Or do you simply want to eat clean, healthy breads?
If the answer was "Yes" to any of the above then you will love my latest book.

Let's face it, bread is a vital part of every person's meal and this cookbook will show you how to bake delicious and nourishing breads that will be in harmony with your digestive system and overall health.

The Heal Your Gut Bread Book caters to several special diets including:

- GLUTEN FREE
- DAIRY FREE
- GAPS (Gut and Psychology Syndrome)

- LEAKY GUT
- LOW CARB
- PALEO

Get your copy now and start baking away!

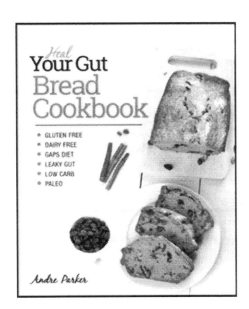

https://www.amazon.com/dp/B06WV98KQL

# TABLE of CONTENTS

# My GAPS Journey

The GAPS diet is life changing, and it has certainly changed my life.

Prior to starting this diet, I suffered from numerous gut health issues. These issues continued for six years before I discovered the GAPS diet.

I had a number of different symptoms which I am sure many of you reading this could relate to. Some of these symptoms included constipation, chronic fatigue, weight gain, sugar addiction, carbohydrate addiction, and I even dealt with two different types of parasites (blastocystis hominis and dientamoeba fragilis). As if you thought this wasn't enough, I also suffered from bacteria imbalances and overgrowth, gastritis, Helicobacter Pylori and ulcerative colitis. After almost each colonoscopy, I also had polyps removed. To say the least, my digestive health was almost nonexistent. Due to the parasites and all the other conditions, I could not absorb any nutrients properly and as a result I was deficient in a number of essential vitamins and minerals.

I had colonoscopies and gastroscopies every year for those six years, and the solution was always the same. The doctor's response was always the same: "Here is a course of heavy antibiotics and off you go, come back next year." Little did I know that conventional medicine was just making me worse, and every course of antibiotics I took just caused more damage to my gut.

I finally gave up on conventional medicine and symptom-based treatments and turned to natural medicine when I came across an excellent naturopath earlier this year that literally changed my life. She had me take every test possible: blood, urine, stool, and discovered the root cause of my problems. I had serious bacteria imbalance in my gut, and two different types of parasites. When she saw all my test results, she just looked at me and said, "No wonder you feel like crap." I finally reached the point where I was sick and tired of feeling tired all the time, and these were my very first steps towards making a huge change in my life.

This particular naturopath suggested that we do a total reset and start again. I did an intracolonic infusion which basically meant inserting a large dose of antibiotics (one last time) into my gut to kill everything! I was then to follow the GAPS diet and like a baby, build up my gut health from scratch. This is where the GAPS diet came into effect.

After being on the GAPS diet for a few months, I returned to my normal healthy weight, and most importantly my symptoms are all gone. Redness and puffiness in my cheeks disappeared. One of the most liberating advantages was just to have regular, normal bowel movements again. People with gut issues understand the pain well.

It's amazing to see how others see a difference in me as well. Everyone comments on how young, and fresh, and even healthy I look, which was definitely not how I was described before. My energy is back and I no longer need 5 cups of coffee to get through my day, and countless sweet and sugary snacks to spike my energy levels. I have never felt better. I attribute all of this to the GAPS diet and the careful guidance from my naturopath. The GAPS diet was my second chance to educate myself and to start again, to heal my body and create a new beginning.

Going through the GAPS diet with the resources available at the time was challenging. The hardest part was the food, especially in the early stages of the diet. It forced me to start learning about food again, and ask myself where does our food come from? Understanding the terms organic, pasture fed, etc. was new to me, and I now had to focus on foods that were deemed to be of highest quality. Since I know this journey can be difficult, I wanted to create an easy-to-follow guide with delicious, nutritious and simple meals. I want to teach you how to get back to the basics and eat the way our parents and grandparents did: wholesome homemade foods using simple techniques.

I would not recommend this diet only for healing ailments, but I would recommend this diet to everyone who wants to achieve optimal gut health and therefore overall health. Health begins in the gut, so we need to establish a strong foundation, and the GAPS diet can help enormously. I would even recommend this diet as a great preventative measure, to help those looking to lose weight and just be healthy. Another reason the GAPS diet comes highly recommended is the fact that this diet not only focuses on strengthening the gut, but also strengthening the gut-brain connection. As it turns out, our gut is home to our "second brain," and this brain actually communicates back and forth with the brain in our head. If our "second brain" is not balanced, we suffer from emotional shifts and even suffer from things like anxiety and depression. The health of our gut impacts our mental health in more ways than you may think, and keeping the gut healthy is the first step in making sure the gut-brain connection is well balanced and operating as it should. Our gut is truly central to the health of our entire body, physically as well as mentally.

I want to say that nothing worthwhile is easy. Seeing as the western diet is so heavily processed and many people have been on this diet all their life, this transition, especially during the GAPS introduction diet, will be hard but the hard work will definitely pay off, I assure you of that. We literally need to start again and rebuild the gut, and this all starts with what we choose to put into our bodies. You have the power to make the choice. Are you going to eat to feed disease or are you going to eat to prevent, heal, and radiate health? Food, healthy, natural, organic, wholesome food, truly is medicine.

If you enjoyed this book,
I'd appreciate it if you would leave a review.

**Simply visit:** https://www.amazon.com/dp/B01MT0X3N3

# Introduction:
## What is the GAPS Diet?

For those of you who have never heard of the GAPS diet, you may be wondering what in the world this diet is all about. You may know that this diet was created as a way to restore gut health, but there is just more to it than that. If the entire diet is somewhat confusing or brand new to you, don't worry. I am going to get down to the basics, and really break down what this diet is all about. Diets are confusing, there's a new one popping up every day, but trust me you won't be confused by the end of this book.

After reading this book, not only will you have a thorough grasp about what the GAPS diet is, but you will be ready to get in the kitchen and start whipping up some delicious recipes to support, nourish, and heal your gut. Let's get started.

First things first, and that's to talk about what the GAPS diet is. GAPS stands for Gut and Psychology Syndrome, and was developed by Dr. Natasha Campbell-McBride MD. The GAPS diet was derived from the SCD (Specific Carbohydrate Diet) as a way to naturally treat inflammatory conditions such as those in the digestive tract. Dr. Campbell took the SCD diet and adjusted it to fit the health care needs of her patients that were suffering from various digestive as well as neurological conditions that resulted from an imbalance in the bacterial ecosystem that lives in the gastrointestinal tract. The new protocol Dr. Campbell would go on to call the GAPS diet focuses on removing foods from the diet that are very difficult to digest, as well as foods that are known to cause damage to the gut flora in your digestive tract. This diet focuses on replacing these gut-depriving and damaging foods with foods that are not only incredibly nutrient-dense but foods that will also allow the intestinal lining of the gut a chance to heal. With intestinal permeability on the rise, it's important to find a diet that is going to focus on the healing aspect of things and focus on foods that are going to give the digestive system the boost that it needs to thrive.

We are going to talk extensively about what foods you should be eating on the GAPS diet to promote a healthy gut in the following section, but it is important to talk about the foods that people should be avoiding on the GAPS diet. Since this diet has such as specific approach to helping neurological as well as digestive conditions, there are very specific foods that are off limits in the GAPS diet. There are also various stages of this diet, where different foods are either allowed into the diet, or not allowed into the diet.

However, no matter what stage of the diet you are in, steering clear of processed foods is essential. There are far too many convenient food options in today's society, and the majority of these convenience foods are highly processed. Many of the foods that are seen today are tampered with, and often times manmade in a lab. Processing of food changes both its chemical as well as biological structure, and it also depletes the food of the nutritional value it may have once had. It's also important not to forget that our bodies were not designed to digest processed foods that have been changed and tampered with from their original state.

There are also chemicals added to processed foods in order to add in flavors and colors that have been lost due to processing. These chemicals have been shown to cause hyperactivity, learning disabilities, among various other health conditions. Our digestive system also takes a massive hit when we consume processed and chemical-laden foods. As stated before, no matter what stage of the GAPS diet you are in, processed foods must be eliminated in order to heal.

Sugar is another food to be eliminated from the diet. Not only is sugar incredibly addictive, but sugar has a very adverse effect on gut flora; this can be terrible for anyone who already suffers from digestive issues. Soya is another major problem. Unfortunately, much of the industry uses genetically modified soya, so it is best to avoid it all together. On top of the genetically modified soya concern, it is also very high in phytates, which are substances that are naturally found in the bran of all grains. The issue with phytates is that they can bind to minerals and then prevent them from being absorbed. Many people following this diet may already be deficient in certain vitamins and minerals, so the last thing you want to do is consume a food that is going to strip your body of the vitamins and minerals that it needs to thrive. Wheat is something else you are going to want to remove from your diet when following the GAPS protocol. Gluten-free diets have been shown to improve symptoms associated with certain conditions such as autism and even schizophrenia, as well as digestive issues. Refined gluten containing carbohydrates such as white bread, white pasta, and other refined products feed parasites as well as harmful bacteria, not to mention fungi in the gut, yuck! For this reason, gluten and wheat products are kept out of the GAPS diet to prevent further damage to an already sensitive and potentially toxin-ridden body. Wheat is also a very common food allergy and sensitivity, so it is best to avoid, especially during the healing process.

We are going to talk much more about what you can and cannot eat when following the GAPS protocol in the sections to come, so don't worry if you are not entirely clear on what you should be avoiding just yet!

I hope that you are starting to get excited about the GAPS diet. This diet completely changed my life, and I am hopeful that GAPS can truly benefit you as well. Let's head over to the next section where I am going to talk about how the GAPS diet may be able to improve your overall health, so you can determine if this is the diet for you.

# How the GAPS Diet Can Benefit You

How can the GAPS diet benefit you? This is the burning question that everyone wants the answer to. What is it about the GAPS diet that makes it stand out from the thousands of other diets available today? The first thing about this diet that makes it different from most is stated quite clearly in the name "GAPS." This diet takes an approach to heal both the gut and the mind, which is genius because more and more research is coming out on the brain-gut connection. Basically, if your gut is imbalanced, your mental health may be as well. This diet takes on a whole new approach to eating, far different than many other diets, something that is incredibly important when you are looking for a new dietary protocol. A whole body approach is necessary to reach complete health, and starting with the gut is the best place to start.

This diet has countless benefits, but one of the primary benefits is obviously its ability to support gut health. For me, the GAPS diet completely transformed the health of my digestive system, and I am living proof that even with a gut that was in a state of disarray, the GAPS diet turned it around for me in just a short amount of time. The GAPS diet is most commonly used for and has shown to be incredibly helpful for those suffering from Irritable Bowel Syndrome, Leaky Gut, autism, ADHD, depression, anxiety, as well as depression. As you can see, the diet helps both psychological conditions as well as physiological issues within the gut. This diet is geared towards repairing the gut wall, rebalancing healthy gut flora, and eliminating and stopping the toxic overload from harmful bacteria that may be found in your gut. GAPS also helps to prevent toxins from entering the bloodstream and focuses on easy-to-digest foods so that your gut, as well as your entire body, can heal.

As you can see, this diet can help to support more than one condition, and even if you don't have any of the issues listed above, or you don't suffer from digestive or psychological imbalances, this diet may still be able to help you. With a focus on extremely high quality foods, and foods to nourish your body, you really can't go wrong by starting the GAPS protocol. There are endless benefits of this diet, and GAPS has allowed me to unleash my potential to feel great and achieve health so that I can live each day with vibrancy for life-exuding health and happiness.

# The Importance of Knowing Where Your Food Comes From

When you sit down at your dinner table, do you know where your food came from? When you enjoy a meal at a restaurant, do you know where that food came from? Chances are the answer is no, as most people simply have no idea where the food on their plate comes from. Sure, you know that your food came from the grocery store, and went from the shelf to your cart, and then to your plate, but knowing where your food comes from before it makes its way onto grocery store shelves is incredibly important. This is a huge component of the GAPS diet. Knowing where your food comes from and understanding how the quality of your food affects your health is something that the GAPS diet puts a huge emphasis on.

Now, if you're anything like me, having to learn about all the different terminology when it comes to food quality was a bit stressful. Having not known the importance of what grass fed, pasture raised, or organic meant to my body meant that this was something I was going to have to put some time into and learn about. I know this can all be confusing which is why I am going to shed some light on first and foremost why knowing where your food comes from is so important.

Knowing where your food comes from is crucial for a number of different reasons. One of the primary reasons for this is the fact that large corporations do not always have your best interest in mind. While you may think that large companies may only create products that are safe for consumption, this may not always be the case. Many large companies choose to put a ton of salt, sugar, and artificial ingredients into their products because this is the fast and easy way to go. It is cheaper to load food products up with the artificial junk as opposed to choosing clean and organic, more expensive ingredients.

Food is also so incredibly processed today. The foods we eat are so refined and lack nutritional value. Since foods are so overly processed and virtually "dead," the large food companies load the products up with a tremendous amount of sugar, especially with corn syrup, just to make it edible. Stick to the natural food options, and avoid the packaged food items. These foods are far from what our body recognizes as "natural."

You will also want to know what animals are fed before you bite into your steak or chicken dinner. Most of what the animals eat, you will be eating too! I remember seeing a quote at my local butchery that read "we are what are our food ate" and it couldn't be truer. Conventionally fed animals are often loaded with steroids, hormones, and antibiotics. Consuming large amounts of commercially fed animal products that have been pumped with loads of antibiotics can eventually make you antibiotic resistant as well, not to mention the harm these antibiotics are doing to your gut bacteria. This is just scraping the surface when it comes to the dangers of consuming conventionally raised animal products. These animals are also fed grains and corn, which is a primary reason the animals get sick in the first place, and then require antibiotic treatment. It turns out that grass-fed cows do not get sick as much as corn-fed cows. Why? Well, because grass is what the cow is supposed to eat. Think of it this way. If we consumed processed and artificial products every single day, we probably wouldn't feel good, and our immune systems would be incredibly weak. Same comes for the animals who consume foods that are so far from what they would naturally eat in the wild. This is just another reason why it's critical to know where your food is coming from. Are you consuming a cow that has been fed corn, or are you consuming animal products that were pasture raised and grass fed? The choice is ultimately up to you to investigate and read the food labels.

Another reason to care about where your food comes from is to avoid GMOs. GMO stands for genetically modified organisms. GMOs are exactly as they sound, genetically modified in a lab. Not only are GMOs bad for your body but they are bad for the farmer and bad for the environment. The health consequences of consuming genetically modified organisms are very unknown, and GMO foods have not been shown to be safe to eat. To be on the safe side, it is best to avoid all GMO products, and the best way to do this is to focus on enjoying all organic foods. If a food is labeled organic, you can rest assured that the food is GMO-free.

Choosing organic products will also help to avoid toxic pesticide and herbicide contamination. Conventional fruits and vegetables are excessively sprayed with pesticides. These chemicals have been known to cause hormonal imbalances, and can even disrupt the digestive system. It is best to choose organic foods.

Lastly, if you do not pay attention to where your food comes from, you may be spending more money on healthcare than food in the long run. Spending a little extra money upfront to pay for high quality organic foods may save you lots of money in the future. We are not going to get healthier by spending less money on food by consuming over-processed, artificial junk. The less we spend on food, the more we spend on healthcare.

The bottom line is that it's essential to pay attention to where your food is coming from. Ask questions when you go out to dinner, ask where the food comes from. Pay attention to food labels, and buy organic whenever possible. When it comes to animal products, opt for grass-fed. By choosing grass-fed products, you can have peace of mind that the animals were not fed an inflammatory diet . Choose pasture-raised as well. When you choose pasture-raised foods, you are opting for animal products that have received a large part of their nutrition from organically managed pasture. If you just choose pasture-raised, the animals may have received a portion of their diet from supplemental organic grains, but when you choose pasture-raised, 100% grass-fed, you are choosing the highest quality available. While it may cost a few extra dollars to buy the quality products, you may end up saving your money and avoiding unnecessary health bills down the road. Invest in your health now, and know where your food comes from. Your body is going to thank you for it in the long run.

# Base Foods for the GAPS Diet

The GAPS diet can be confusing to some, especially because there are a number of different stages within the diet. The purpose of this book is to clear up any of that confusion and make it easy for you to jump in and get started on transforming your health. This is where this chapter comes in. Even though there are different stages of the GAPS diet, there are some base foods that you should keep on hand that are commonly seen in more than one stage of the GAPS diet.

To get started, you will want to stock up on stock! A large part of the GAPS diet focuses on making homemade stock, so you will definitely want to make a big batch before you fully get started on the diet. You can even make many pots of stock to make sure that you are well prepared, as bone broth and homemade stocks are going to be your primary source of fuel early on in the diet. Get your mason jars out, or pick a few inexpensive ones up at the store so that you can easily store the broth in the fridge. Store a few jars in the refrigerator, and the rest in a freezer-safe container. Don't be shy here, make a ton! You will be enjoying your delicious homemade stock at every meal early on, so you will probably need more than you initially think.

The next things to stock up on are veggies. You will want to get lots of vegetables to add to your soups! Some of the GAPS-approved vegetables include broccoli, bok choy, carrots, cauliflower, collard greens, spinach, garlic, kale, winter squash, and turnips. These veggies are approved so long as they are cooked, and enjoyed in your stock.

Next, stock up on sauerkraut. Sauerkraut is a fermented food that is excellent for promoting digestion, and something that you will be able to enjoy during different stages of the GAPS diet. You will want to make your own sauerkraut which takes a few days, so starting early is key. Check out the recipe section for an easy homemade sauerkraut recipe that will quickly become a staple in your diet.

There are many different foods to enjoy as part of the GAPS diet, but having these foods ready and available before you even start the diet will set you up for success! These foods are easy to make, inexpensive, and store well so stock up now, and you will thank yourself later!

# Necessary Equipment

As with any diet, kitchen equipment certainly comes in handy! While this is not something to stress about, prepping your kitchen before you start the GAPS diet can be very helpful, and can help to keep you on track in the long term.

Since the GAPS diet is a major change for most people, not everyone may have the necessary equipment, and that's okay. Slow and steady wins the race, and slowly stocking your kitchen with the equipment is a great approach.

I have listed some of the things you may want to purchase before starting this diet to make things that much easier. The items listed here are meant to help you cook from scratch. Since not everyone cooks from home as much as this diet recommends, you may find that you don't have everything on this list. Please keep in mind that these are just recommendations, and again, please do not stress if you don't have everything on the list! This is not meant to make you overwhelmed; it's simply to help ease you into this diet so that you can ultimately achieve success!

## GAPS Diet Kitchen Equipment:

- **Stainless Steel Stock Pot:** A stainless steel stock pot will come in handy when it comes time to making homemade bone broth and stock. I personally use All-Clad but any brand of stainless steel pot will work.
- **Freezer-Safe Jars & Bags:** Prepping your meals while following the GAPS diet will make your life so much less stressful! Having freezer space as well as freezer-safe containers available at all times will come in handy.
- **Juicer:** This is optional, but may come in handy when it comes to stage 4 of the GAPS diet. At stage 4 you can start introducing fresh-pressed juices. You can find juicers as inexpensive as $40 and as expensive as a couple of thousand dollars! It all depends on how much you want to splurge. The lower end juicers should work just fine for the basic GAPS juices.
- **Crockpot:** Cooking with a crockpot can make cooking so much easier! You can even cook bone broth and stock in a crockpot which helps reduce your workload. You can also cook some of your meat products in a crockpot which makes the end product super tender. Cooking your meals in a crockpot has also been shown to help improve the digestibility of the foods which is essential for when you have a sluggish digestive system.

- **Mason Jars:** These jars come in handy for when you are making fermented foods. If you really enjoy making fermented foods, as you will grow to love while following the GAPS diet, purchasing a fermenting crock may be worth the investment.
- **Water Filter:** Knowing what's in your water is just as important as knowing what's in your food. You will want to invest in a good water filter to filter out the impurities found in tap water. Reverse osmosis filters are the best, but if that is out of the budget, you may also want to look into an under-the-sink carbon filter. Keep in mind that there is no evidence that proves that bottled water is any better than tap water, so purchasing a quality water filter will be well worth the investment.

Even if you don't have any of the items on the list, that's okay! Start slow, and get what you can. Focus on getting the essentials such as a high-quality water filter, and at least a crockpot. Having these two things handy will at least ensure that you are drinking pure and clean water and that you have a crockpot to make your broths and stews, which are an essential part of the GAPS diet.

Now that we have your kitchen prepped, head over the next chapter where I share some staple pantry and ingredient items to help get you started.

# Staple Ingredients & Pantry Items

Now that you have your kitchen stocked with the kitchen equipment you need to make all of the wonderful and nourishing recipes on the GAPS diet, let's talk about how to stock your pantry for success, and how to give your kitchen a GAPS detox before you get going.

An important part of starting this diet is cleaning out your kitchen and removing any tempting foods. When you first start the GAPS diet, it may be a bit challenging as your body starts to adjust and the last things you want to have are temptations all around your kitchen, getting in the way of your healing and success with this diet. Before you even head to the grocery store to pick up some staple food items, let's talk about some ways you can detoxify your kitchen.

The first things you will need to eliminate are gluten-containing products. Gluten is not something you will find following the GAPS diet, and something that can cause significant damage to not only your digestive system but your overall health as well. Toss the gluten as well as any other known food allergens. You will also want to read the food labels on all of the foods in your kitchen and toss anything that contains artificial ingredients. You may even want to eliminate kitchen utensils that have been contaminated with things like gluten and known allergens.

Next, deep clean your kitchen! Clean the countertops, your kitchen table, and even the fridge and the freezer. Get everything squeaky clean so that you have a fresh start and reduce the risk of possible contamination as you begin your healing journey. The last tip I have for detoxifying your kitchen is to designate one cabinet, or one area of your fridge or freezer to only contain what you are allowed to have for the introduction stage to this diet. If you eliminate the foods that you are not allowed to have, you have a better chance of having them be out of sight, out of mind. The goal is to set yourself up for as much success as you can so that you will be well on your way to healing your digestive system, and feel better in no time.

So, now that we have your kitchen stocked, detoxed, and ready to go, it's time to make a grocery list and head to the grocery store.

You will want to stock your pantry with items that will frequently be seen throughout the course of this diet, but initially, you may want to prep your kitchen for the introductory foods first. I will talk all about the foods that are acceptable for the GAPS stages 1–6, and lastly the full GAPS diet, but for now, here are some of the staple foods you may want to keep on hand.

- Organic pastured meat
- Organic pastured meat bones
- Organic vegetables
- Nuts (you will be soaking and dehydrating these)
- Raw milk
- Water kefir grains  (these help ferment juice and coconut water into kefir)
- Dairy kefir grains (these ferment milk into kefir)
- Coconut oil
- Raw & local honey
- Free-range organic eggs
- Fermented cod liver oil

Head over to the next chapter where I will break down each stage of the GAPS diet for you so that you know what to stock your kitchen with, what's allowed and what's off limits.

# The GAPS Introduction Diet

## (Stages 1-6)

As you have probably gathered by now, each stage of the GAPS diet allows for different foods. Don't get overwhelmed by this; I am going to make it very easy to follow so that you can feel prepared to tackle this diet, and feel confident in knowing that you are healing your gut in the best possible way that you can.

To start, let's talk about Stage 1 of the GAPS diet. This is the stage where you are most restricted, and you will likely find to be the most challenging. This is because you are probably coming off of a diet that may have been loaded with foods that did not sit well with your body. Starting the GAPS diet may lead to some detox symptoms where you feel intense cravings at times. The grass is truly greener on the other side, so please stick to it. The introduction diet if done right will keep you very well nourished and hydrated which is exactly what your body needs during the adjustment period. To set yourself up for success, it's best to prep a couple of homemade stocks ahead of time, and to be prepared with lots of GAPS-approved vegetables before you get started. This way you can grab and go, and it doesn't take ages to put your meals together. Stage 1 is a very basic diet and consists of the following foods:

## Introduction Diet: Stage 1

- Homemade stock
- Meats & fish cooked into the stock such as:
    - Beef
    - Lamb
    - Chicken
    - Turkey
    - Fish
- Non-fibrous vegetables cooked in the stock, these can include:
    - Collard greens
    - Eggplant
    - Bok choy
    - Kale
    - Spinach

16

- o Zucchini
- o Pumpkin
- o Winter squash
- o Onion
- o Garlic
- o Carrots
- o Broccoli
- o Cauliflower
- o Fermented vegetable juice
- o Turnips

Please note that if you're suffering from extreme cases of diarrhea, it is recommended that you exclude vegetables first, and to focus on stock with probiotic-rich foods every hour, and well-cooked meats as well as fish. You will not want to introduce vegetables until after the diarrhea begins to calm down. You want to reduce that inflammation before adding in the fiber.

- Fermented yogurt & dairy. Only include a small amount each day, about one to two teaspoons, and then gradually work your way up to a tablespoon or so after about five days. Only include fermented yogurt if you are not sensitive or allergic to dairy. Homemade is best, and you can find a homemade recipe in the recipe section of this book. You may also want to consider adding in some whey, sour cream, kefir, or raw milk if you do not have a sensitivity to dairy. Again, quality is key here, so you will want to opt for the highest quality possible. This may be a great option for those who suffer from diarrhea.
- Other fermented foods. There are other ways to get probiotic-rich foods into your diet. The juice from your homemade sauerkraut or fermented vegetables is an excellent option. Try adding these to your soup for an extra probiotic-rich boost. These are the best fermented options if you suffer from constipation.
- Ginger, mint or chamomile tea. You can sweeten your tea with a small amount of raw and local honey if desired. Be sure to use the whole leaf version of tea, and not the powdered version.

The GAPS introduction diet focuses on nourishing foods that nourish the gut lining with things like amino acids, fats, vitamins, and minerals. The foods help to renew the gut lining. The introduction part of the GAPS diet also initially removes any fiber as well as other substances which may cause irritation to the gut which could ultimately interfere with the healing process. Not everyone knows that they have inflammation in the gut, so by focusing on the nourishing and supporting foods, the gut is allowed to heal even in cases where inflammation has gone undetected. The GAPS introduction diet also includes probiotic-rich, healthy bacteria right from the get go so the gut can start repairing itself and heal with beneficial bacteria.

Once the introduction phase of this diet begins, you can decide to move through the diet as fast as your body permits. You may wish to stay at different stages for different periods of time. For example, you may want to only stay on the introduction diet for three days while you stay at the second stage for 4–5 days. Listen to your body, and move through as quickly as you feel is best. The most important thing to remember is to take the introduction diet seriously, and not to skip it. The introduction phase of the GAPS diet is integral to success, and by following this part of the diet, you allow your digestive system to begin the healing process quicker than you would if you completely skipped over it. Stick to the introduction diet for a few days to help improve symptoms before moving to the next stage.

## Stage 2:

You have made it to Stage 2; you are probably hoping that you can add a bit more into your diet! If you've made it to this stage, you are also probably starting to feel better, and are starting to get excited about the amazing possibilities this diet has to heal your gut. Or you've had some detoxifying symptoms or "die-off" and this is great as well because it is a sign that your body is getting rid of the toxins and getting better. For Stage 2, you will still want to be enjoying your soups boiled with meats, veggies, and probiotic-rich foods. You may even want to be enjoying some ginger tea at this point and will want to add some raw organic eggs into the soups. It's important to only add the egg yolks into the soups, removing the egg whites. You can start with one egg yolk per day, and then gradually increase until you are enjoying an egg for each bowl of soup you enjoy. Stick with organic free-range eggs, and only include them if you do not have a sensitivity or allergy to eggs. At this stage, you can also add in some stews and casseroles made with meats and veggies, but avoid any spices in Stage 2. You can, however, add in some sea salt and fresh herbs to spice up the flavor and add in some extra health benefits. You will also want to continue to increase the amount of homemade whey, sour cream, yogurt or kefir in your diet as well as the juice from your homemade sauerkraut and fermented vegetables. You can also add in one small piece of fermented fish per day in Stage 2 such as Swedish gravlax. Homemade ghee can be introduced here at one teaspoon per day and then gradually increased.

## Stage 3:

Welcome to Stage 3! You have started adding more foods into your diet, as you steadily increase the amount of probiotic-rich foods in your diet as well. In Stage 3 you will want to continue with the foods you have been eating, and you can now add a ripe avocado mashed into your soups. Start with about 1–3 teaspoons per day. You can now even add in GAPS-approved pancakes at this stage made from nut butter, eggs, and squash or zucchini! You can find a recipe in the recipe section to get started. You may also start making scrambled eggs cooked in ghee or pork fat, and served with avocado and even some cooked onion. Lastly, start to actually eat the fermented vegetables and sauerkraut instead of only enjoying the juice. Start small and work your way up to having 1–4 teaspoons at each meal.

## Stage 4:

At Stage 4, you will want to gradually increase cooked meats by roasting and grilling them instead of only cooking them in your soups. Enjoy cooked meats with cooked vegetables as well as sauerkraut. You can also now begin enjoying freshly-pressed juice by starting with a very small amount of carrot juice. Once you are comfortable having a full cup per day, you can branch out and try celery, cabbage, lettuce, and mint juices as well. At Stage 4 you are also welcome to add in cold-pressed olive oil, working your way up to 1–2 tablespoons for each meal. Lastly, you can start to bake with ground almonds by making almond bread or make the bread with any other nuts and seeds ground into flour. Check out the bread recipes in the recipe section of this book.

## Stage 5:

In Stage 5 of the GAPS diet, you will want to continue to enjoy all of the nourishing foods you have already added into your diet, and you can begin to add cooked apple puree. Keep an eye out for a recipe in the recipe section! You may also begin adding raw vegetables starting with the softer parts of lettuce and cucumber. Increase until well tolerated, and if diarrhea comes back, you know your body is not quite ready to introduce these foods yet. If the vegetable juices have been well tolerated, you can now begin to add fruits such as pineapple and mango, but still keep citrus fruits out of the recipes at this point.

## Stage 6:

You have almost completed the GAPS introduction diet! I hope that you are feeling so much better and are ready to start the full GAPS diet. For the sixth stage, if all of the other foods have been well tolerated, you can now try some raw apple with the skin peeled, and slowly introduce raw fruits with a little bit more honey in your diet as well. You can also introduce baked goodies that are GAPS approved, which you will find in the recipe section of this book. For baked goods, you will want to stick to dried fruit as the sweetener.

While it may seem like six stages are quite a lot to get through, I hope that breaking down each stage makes things a little more clear. As you can see, each stage builds on each other, and goes at a slow pace as not to trigger any inflammation in your body. It's also important to rotate each food seen in each stage. As you progress through the diet, remember to keep enjoying the foods from the previous stage as well so you are gradually increasing the amount of food you are eating. Listen to your body, and go at a pace that works for you. Once you are finished with all six stages, you are ready for the full GAPS diet which we will be talking about in the next chapter!

# The Full GAPS Diet

Now that you know what stages 1–6 look like, are you ready to learn about what the full GAPS diet entails? The full GAPS diet is something that, once you become accustomed to it, will likely become a staple in your diet long term. The GAPS diet is known to help people feel ten times better than before they started the diet.

Once you start this phase of this diet, you will be very experienced with the GAPS way of eating, and you will probably be feeling so much better! You will also have gained some insight as to how your body responds to certain foods. Keeping a food diary can be very helpful, especially during the introduction diet; this way you can reference back to this when you start the full diet. This will help you pinpoint which foods agree with you and which do not.

The full GAPS diet, once started, will need to be followed for about two years. While two years is recommended, some may stay on the diet more than two years, and some less. Some people who may have milder conditions may be able to start introducing non-allowed foods after one year, while others will have to strictly stick to the diet for much longer. It all depends on your individual case. The general rule of thumb is to stick to the GAPS diet in its entirety for two years before you start adding in non-GAPS approved foods.

A typical full GAPS diet would look something like this: You would start your day with a glass of filtered water with either a slice of lemon or a teaspoon of apple cider vinegar. You can then enjoy a glass of fresh pressed fruit or vegetable juice. This is where the investment in a juicer comes in handy! For breakfast, you can choose eggs with sausage and vegetables and some onions or even a GAPS-approved homemade muffin. For lunch, a homemade soup with some probiotic-rich foods would be great, and lastly, dinner could include a homemade stew or any meat or fish cooked with vegetables.

Stick to this diet for at least two years or longer if you would like to help heal your gut and promote overall wellness. Keep in mind that getting off of the GAPS diet could lead to unwanted reactions if done suddenly, and you need to have 6 months or more of normal digestion before you even consider adding in non-GAPS foods. Sticking to the GAPS diet will also prevent you from consuming a modern diet packed with sugar and processed foods again, which is not a bad thing! Your body will become accustomed to eating the foods it's meant to, which is why adding in the processed junk could potentially cause you to feel quite ill.

Keep in mind that starting the GAPS diet is incredibly rewarding for your overall health, and one of the best decisions you can make for your gut health!

If you are ready to get started on your GAPS journey, head to the next section where I share 30 delicious GAPS recipes for every stage.

# 50 RECIPES

## TO NOURISH & REPAIR

# GAPS STAGE 1

# Ginger Chamomile Tea

**Serves: 1**
**Prep Time:** 5 minutes
**Cooking Time:** 5 minutes

## Ingredients:

1 Tbsp. chamomile flowers
¼ tsp. freshly grated ginger
1 tsp. freshly squeezed lemon juice

## Directions:

1. Add all of the ingredients to a cup, pour in 8 ounces of boiling water, and steep for five minutes.
2. Strain, and enjoy.

# GAPS Chicken Stock

**Serves:** 8
**Prep Time:** 10 minutes
**Cooking Time:** 2 hours

## Ingredients:

1 whole organic chicken
1 pinch of Celtic sea salt
Filtered water

## Directions:

1. Simply add the chicken to the base of a large pot, and fill with water. Add enough water to cover the chicken.
2. Add a pinch of salt, and simmer for 2 hours covered.
3. Once cooked, remove the chicken, and run the stock through a thin sieve.
4. Store in mason jars in the refrigerator or freezer.
5. Strip off the soft tissues from the bones to later use in soups.

# GAPS Beef Stock

**Serves:** 8
**Prep Time:** 10 minutes
**Cooking Time:** 2 hours

## Ingredients:

6 beef soup bones
1 tsp. apple cider vinegar
1 pinch of Celtic sea salt
Filtered water

## Directions:

1. Simply add the beef soup bones to the base of a large crock pot and fill with water. Add enough water to cover the beef bones.
2. Add a pinch of salt and the apple cider vinegar. Turn the crock pot on high and as soon as the stock starts to simmer, turn to low.
3. Keep it at a low simmer for 12–24 hours.
4. Once the stock is cooked, strain and add to mason jars.
5. Store in mason jars in the refrigerator or freezer.

# Homemade Yogurt

**Serves:** 8
**Prep Time:** 10 minutes +
fermentation time
**Cooking Time:** 0 minutes

## Ingredients:

½ gallon organic milk (grass-fed is best)
1 packet yogurt starter culture

## Directions:

1. Start by pouring the milk into a large pot over low heat. Stir and heat until the milk reaches about 180°F.
2. Allow the milk to cool, and then remove one cup of the milk and place into a mixing bowl with the yogurt starter packet. (If the packet requires more or less milk, follow the packet instructions.)
3. Stir the cultured milk into the pot with the rest of the milk. Evenly distribute the mixture into mason jars.
4. Place the yogurt into the oven with the oven lights on. Do not actually turn your oven heat on though. Allow the yogurt to sit in the oven for 24 hours. Remove the yogurt, and place in the refrigerator to set.
5. Enjoy once set, and serve with a drizzle of honey if desired.

## Cooking Tips:

Alternatively, you can set a dehydrator to 105°F and let the yogurt sit undisturbed in the dehydrator for 24 hours. You can also use a yogurt maker or allow the yogurt to sit someplace warm between 105–113°F, such as on top of your broiler.

# Homemade Kefir

**Makes: 1 quart**
**Prep Time:** 10 minutes +
fermentation time
**Cooking Time:** 0 minutes

## Ingredients:

1 quart of raw milk
1 Tbsp. dairy kefir grains

## Directions:

1. Start by placing the milk kefir grains at the bottom of a large mason jar. You can use two and split the kefir grains if necessary.
2. Pour the raw milk over the grains.
3. Cover the mason jars with the lid, but do not tighten the lid. Allow the kefir to sit out and culture for 24 hours, less time if you want a thinner consistency. You can allow the kefir to sit in a warm place between 105–113°F. This can be in a yogurt maker, or on top of your broiler.
4. Strain the milk kefir into a new mason jar, cover and place in the refrigerator.
5. You can make a new batch right away, or allow your kefir grains to sit in a bath of water for a few days before using them again.

# Sauerkraut Juice

**Serves: 18**
**Prep Time:** 10 minutes +
fermentation time
**Cooking Time:** 0 minutes

## Ingredients:

1 head of cabbage
2 Tbsp. Celtic sea salt
Filtered water

## Directions:

1. Start by chopping the head of cabbage in a food processor or high-speed blender. You will want to cut the cabbage into smaller pieces before blending.
2. Transfer the chopped cabbage into a large mixing bowl, and sprinkle with the salt. Allow this to sit for one hour.
3. Take a couple of large mason jars, fill them ⅓ of the way full with the salted cabbage, and then fill the rest with the filtered water, leaving a little room at the top.
4. Cover the jars and allow them to sit for 7–14 days on the countertop.
5. After the fermentation process, store in the fridge, and use the juice in the first stage of the GAPS diet, and the actual sauerkraut in the following stages.

## Cooking Tips:

If you want to enjoy sauerkraut juice sooner than 7–14 days, you can use a starter culture in place of the salt. If using a high-quality starter culture, you will be able to enjoy your sauerkraut within 5 days as opposed to up to two weeks.

# Mint Tea

**Serves: 1**
**Prep Time:** 5 minutes
**Cooking Time:** 5 minutes

## Ingredients:

1 Tbsp. fresh mint leaves
8 ounces of hot filtered water
½ tsp. raw honey

## Directions:

1. Place the mint leaves in a tea pot with the hot water.
2. Steep for 5 minutes before straining.
3. Sweeten with raw honey, and enjoy right away.

# GAPS Fish Stock

**Makes: 4 quarts**
**Prep Time:** 10 minutes
**Cooking Time:** 1 ½ hours.

## Ingredients:

2 non-oily pieces of wild-caught fish
4 quarts of filtered water
1 tsp. Celtic sea salt

## Directions:

1. Add the whole fish to a large stock pot, cover with the water and season with salt.
2. Simmer for 1 ½ hours.
3. Once cooked, strain, and remove the soft tissue from the fish to use in later soups.

# GAPS STAGE 2

# Chicken Stock Vegetable Soup

**Prep Time:** 20 minutes
**Cooking Time:** 20 minutes
**Serves:** 1

## Ingredients:

1 cup of GAPS chicken stock
2 Tbsp. chopped onion
1 carrot, chopped
1 celery stalk, chopped
1 tsp. freshly chopped thyme

## Directions:

1. Add the chicken stock to a large stock pot over medium heat and bring to a boil.
2. Add the remaining ingredients minus the thyme, and bring to a simmer.
3. Simmer for 20 minutes, and then serve with fresh thyme.

# Creamy Cauliflower Soup

**Prep Time:** 10 minutes
**Cooking Time:** 10 minutes
**Serves: 1**

## Ingredients:

1 cup of GAPS chicken stock
¾ cup of cauliflower florets
1 garlic clove, chopped
¼ of an onion, chopped
1 Tbsp. sauerkraut juice
½ tsp. Celtic sea salt
1 tsp. freshly chopped chives

## Directions:

1. Start by placing the cauliflower and the chicken stock into a stock pot and bring to a boil.
2. Add the remaining ingredients, and simmer for 10 minutes.
3. Using an immersion blender or high-speed blender, blend until smooth.
4. Garnish with chopped chives.

# Sage & Pumpkin Soup

**Prep Time:** 10 minutes
**Cooking Time:** 25 minutes
**Serves: 4**

## Ingredients:

4 cups homemade pumpkin puree
6 cups of homemade GAPS chicken stock
1 garlic clove, chopped
1 onion, chopped
4 Tbsp. homemade ghee (if tolerated)
1 tsp. Celtic sea salt
1 tsp. dried sage
Cilantro for serving (Optional)

## Directions:

1. Start by heating a large stock pot over medium heat with the ghee. Add the garlic, onion, and sage, and sauté for 5 minutes.
2. Add the remaining ingredients, and simmer for 20 minutes or until the squash (I'm thinking this should be pumpkin here as this is what is in the ingredient list, not squash) is tender.
3. Using an immersion blender or high-speed blender, blend until smooth.
4. Garnish with cilantro if desired, and enjoy right away.
5. Store any leftovers in the fridge or freezer.

# Lemon Chicken Soup

**Prep Time:** 10 minutes
**Cooking Time:** 25 minutes
**Serves: 1**

## Ingredients:

3 organic chicken thighs (skin-on and bone-in)
1 cup of homemade GAPS chicken stock
1 garlic clove, chopped
1 Tbsp. chopped onion
1 Tbsp. ghee (If tolerated)
1 tsp. Celtic sea salt
½ tsp. fresh dill for garnish
1 slice of lemon

## Directions:

1. Start by heating a large stock pot over medium heat with the ghee. Add the garlic and onion, and sauté for 3 minutes.
2. Add the remaining ingredients minus the dill and simmer for 20 minutes or until the chicken is cooked through.
3. Once cooked, remove the skin and meat from the chicken and mix the meat into the soup. Stir to combine. (You can keep the bones to make bone broth.)
4. Garnish with dill.

# Herbed Chicken Soup

**Prep Time:** 20 minutes
**Cooking Time:** 30 minutes
**Serves:** 4

## Ingredients:

1 lb. cubed chicken breast, cubed
4 cups of homemade GAPS chicken stock
1 garlic clove, chopped
½ cup chopped tomatoes
½ cup chopped celery
1 zucchini, chopped
1 tsp. Celtic sea salt
1 tsp. fresh thyme
½ tsp. dried oregano
1 Tbsp. fresh basil, chopped
1 Tbsp. homemade ghee

## Directions:

1. Start by heating a large stock pot over medium heat with the ghee. Add in the garlic, and chicken, and sauté until browned.
2. Add in the remaining ingredients, and bring to a boil.
3. Simmer for 20-25 minutes or until the squash, and zucchini is super tender.
4. Enjoy right away!

# Butternut Squash Soup

**Prep Time:** 20 minutes
**Cooking Time:** 30 minutes
**Serves: 4**

## Ingredients:

1 butternut squash peeled, seeded, and cubed
3 cups of homemade GAPS chicken stock
1 yellow onion, chopped
½ cup of chopped carrots
1 tsp. Celtic sea salt
1 egg yolk (optional)

## Directions:

1. Simply add all of the ingredients minus the egg yolk to a large stock pot, and bring to a boil.
2. Simmer for 30–35 minutes or until the butternut squash is tender. Add the egg yolk at the end of cooking, and stir.
3. Using an immersion blender or a high-speed blender, blend until super smooth.
4. Enjoy right away, and store the leftovers in the fridge or freezer.

# Gut Healing Chicken Stew

**Prep Time:** 20 minutes
**Cooking Time:** 8 hours
**Serves:** 8

## Ingredients:

2 pounds of organic pasture-raised chicken thighs (skin-on & bone-in)
Homemade GAPS chicken stock (enough to cover the chicken thighs)
1 zucchini, peeled, seeded, and chopped
4 carrots, chopped
1 cup of chopped mushrooms
3 tomatoes, peeled, seeded, and chopped
¼ cup fresh parsley
1 Tbsp. fresh thyme, chopped
1 tsp. Celtic sea salt

## Directions:

1. Add all of the ingredients to a large stock pot, and cover with chicken stock.
2. Bring to a boil, and then cook on low for 8 hours or until the chicken is thoroughly cooked, and the vegetables are tender.
3. Once cooked, remove the skin and meat from the chicken and mix the meat into the vegetables. Stir to combine. (You can keep the bones to make bone broth.)
4. Enjoy.

# Gut Healing Beef Stew

**Prep Time:** 20 minutes
**Cooking Time:** 8 hours
**Serves:** 8

## Ingredients:

2 organic beef soup bones, with meat
4 cups homemade GAPS beef stock
4 cloves of garlic, chopped
1 yellow onion, chopped
1 zucchini, chopped
2 Tbsp. ghee
1 tsp. Celtic sea salt

## Directions:

1. Add all of the ingredients minus the zucchini to a crock pot or slow cooker, and cook on low for 6 hours.
2. During the last 2 hours of cooking, add the zucchini.
3. Once cooked, remove the meat from the bones and mix the meat into the stew. Stir to combine. (You can keep the bones to make bone broth.)
4. Enjoy.

# Squash Casserole

**Prep Time:** 20 minutes
**Cooking Time:** 40 minutes
**Serves:** 8

## Ingredients:

2 lbs. of organic pasture-raised chicken, cubed
4 zucchini, peeled, seeded, and chopped
¾ cups GAPS chicken stock
1 Tbsp. ghee
1 tsp. oregano
1 tsp. chopped chives
1 tsp. Celtic sea salt

## Directions:

1. Start by preheating the oven to 350°F, and greasing a roasting pan.
2. Add the stock to the bottom of the roasting pan, and then add the chicken. Season with salt, and oregano.
3. Add the zucchini to top the chicken.
4. Top with the chopped chives.
5. Cover the pan with foil, and bake for 40–45 minutes or until the chicken is thoroughly cooked through.

# Homemade Ghee

**Prep Time:** 20 minutes
**Cooking Time:** 40 minutes
**Makes: 1 pound of ghee**

## Ingredients:

1 pound of unsalted high-quality organic butter

## Directions:

1. Start by preheating the oven to 250°F.
2. Add the butter to an oven safe dish, and bake for about an hour, checking at the 40-minute mark making sure the butter does not burn.
3. Carefully remove the dish and pour the brownish fat off the top, leaving the remaining solid part in the dish.
4. Store the ghee in a glass mason jar.

# Butternut Squash & Meatball Casserole

**Prep Time:** 20 minutes
**Cooking Time:** 45 minutes
**Serves: 4**

## Ingredients:

1 pound of grass-fed ground beef
1 clove of garlic, chopped
1 1/2 cups of GAPS beef stock
1 medium butternut squash, peeled and chopped
1 tsp. fresh parsley, chopped
1 tsp. fresh thyme
½ tsp. Celtic sea salt

## Directions:

1. Start by preheating the oven to 400°F, and greasing the bottom of a roasting pan.
2. Add the ground beef and herbs to a large mixing bowl, and stir to combine. Form into meatballs.
3. Place the cubed squash in the bottom of the greased baking dish. Pour the broth to cover the squash, adding more if necessary. Top with the meatballs.
4. Bake for 45 minutes or until the meatballs are brown and the squash is tender.
5. Season with salt, and enjoy.

# STAGE 3

# Hazelnut Pancakes

**Prep Time:** 10 minutes
**Cooking Time:** 15 minutes
**Serves:** 4

## Ingredients:

1 cup of cooked butternut squash
½ cup of homemade hazelnut butter (see recipe on the following page)
4 organic pasture-raised eggs
Ghee for cooking
1 tsp. of raw honey per serving if tolerated.

## Directions:

1. Start by warming a large pan over low to medium heat with the ghee.
2. While the pan is heating up, add the squash and hazelnut butter to a food processor, and process until smooth.
3. Next, add the eggs and process again until combined.
4. Add about 2 tablespoons of the batter to the pre-greased warm pan, and cook until the bottom starts to brown. Flip and cook for another minute or so on the other side or until the pancake starts to firm up a bit.
5. Serve with extra ghee, and a drizzle of honey if tolerated or if desired.

# Hazelnut Butter

**Prep Time:** 20 minutes
**Cooking Time:** 0 minutes
**Makes: About 2 cups**

## Ingredients:

3 cups of raw organic hazelnuts
½ tsp Celtic sea salt
1 tsp. cinnamon
1 Tbsp. raw honey

## Directions:

1. Start by removing the skin on the hazelnuts.
2. Once the skin is removed, transfer to a food processor and process until the nuts create a smooth and creamy nut butter consistency. Add the cinnamon, raw honey, and salt, and process again.
3. Store in mason jars, and store in the fridge to help maintain freshness.

# Almond Butter

**Prep Time:** 20 minutes
**Cooking Time:** 0 minutes
**Makes: About 2 cups**

## Ingredients:

3 cups of raw organic almonds
½ cup of coconut oil, warmed
1 tsp. cinnamon
1 Tbsp. raw honey
1 tsp. Celtic sea salt

## Directions:

1. Start by adding the almonds, salt, and cinnamon to a food processor and blend until an almond flour forms.
2. Add the coconut oil and raw honey, and process until an almond butter consistency forms.
3. Store in mason jars, and store in the fridge to help maintain freshness.

# Avocado Eggs

**Prep Time:** 10 minutes
**Cooking Time:** 10 minutes
**Serves:** 1

## Ingredients:

2 organic pasture-raised eggs
¼ of a cup cubed organic avocado
1 Tbsp. chopped white onion
1 Tbsp. chopped celery
1 Tbsp. chopped carrots
1 tsp. sauerkraut (See recipe)
1 Tbsp. ghee for cooking

## Directions:

1. Start by heating a large skillet over medium heat with the ghee.
2. While the pan is heating, whisk together the eggs with the chopped onion, celery, and carrots.
3. Add the eggs to the warmed pan, and scramble. Sauté until well cooked.
4. Serve the eggs with a side of cubed avocado, and topped with sauerkraut.

# Cauliflower Mash

**Prep Time:** 10 minutes
**Cooking Time:** 10 minutes
**Serves:** 6

## Ingredients:

1 head of organic cauliflower, cut into florets
4 cups of homemade GAPS chicken stock
¼ cup of homemade ghee
1 tsp. Celtic sea salt

## Directions:

1. Start by adding the cauliflower and the stock to a large stock pot, and bring to a boil. Boil for 7–8 minutes or until tender.
4. Add the salt and ghee, and with an immersion blender, blend until smooth. Alternatively, you can add the mixture to a food processor or high-speed blender and blend until smooth.
5. Enjoy while warm.

# Garlic & Cauliflower Soup

**Prep Time:** 10 minutes
**Cooking Time:** 25 minutes
**Serves: 4**

## Ingredients:

1 head of organic cauliflower, cut into florets
4 cloves of garlic
1 onion, chopped
1 celery stalk, chopped
6 Tbsp. homemade ghee
1 tsp. dried basil
1 tsp. thyme
1 tsp. Celtic sea salt
4 cups of GAPS chicken stock

## Directions:

1. Add all of the ingredients to a large stock pot, and bring to a boil. Simmer for 25 minutes or until the cauliflower is tender.
2. With an immersion blender, blend until smooth. Alternatively, you can add the mixture to a food processor or high-speed blender and blend until smooth.

# Breakfast Egg Burrito

**Prep Time:** 10 minutes
**Cooking Time:** 10 minutes
**Serves:** 1

## Ingredients:

2 organic pasture-raised eggs
¼ lb. of grass-fed ground beef
¼ of an onion, chopped
¼ cup cubed avocado
½ cup of GAPS beef broth
1 Tbsp. homemade ghee
1 tsp. Celtic sea salt

## Directions:

1. Start by heating a large skillet over medium heat with the ghee. Add the beef broth and the ground beef to the skillet, and sauté until well cooked. This should take about 7–10 minutes.
2. While the ground beef is cooking, whisk the eggs with the chopped onion, and add to another skillet with ghee. Cook on one side until the eggs start to firm up a bit. Add the ground beef to one half of the egg mix along with the avocado and salt. Flip one half of the egg mixture over, and cook for another 5 minutes.
3. Enjoy right away and serve with a diced tomato if desired.

# Broccoli Soup

**Prep Time:** 10 minutes
**Cooking Time:** 20 minutes
**Serves: 4**

## Ingredients:

2 heads of broccoli, cut into florets
1 white onion, chopped
4 cups of GAPS chicken stock
½ cup of homemade ghee
1 tsp. ground cinnamon
1 tsp. Celtic sea salt

## Directions:

1. Add all of the ingredients to a large stock pot, and bring to a boil. Simmer for 25 minutes or until the broccoli is tender.
3. With an immersion blender, blend until smooth. Alternatively, you can add the mixture to a food processor or high-speed blender and blend until smooth.

# STAGE 4

# Almond Flour

**Prep Time:** 10 minutes
**Cooking Time:** 0 minutes
**Makes: About 3 cups**

## Ingredients:

3 cups of blanched almonds

## Directions:

1. Simply place the almonds into a high-speed blender or food processor, and blend until a fine powder is formed.
2. Use to make GAPS-approved baked goods.

# Almond Bread

**Prep Time:** 10 minutes
**Cooking Time:** 40 minutes
**Serves:** 16

## Ingredients:

2 ½ cups homemade almond flour
3 organic pasture-raised eggs
¼ cup homemade ghee
½ cup homemade yogurt
1 tsp. ground cinnamon

## Directions:

1. Start by preheating the oven to 350°F, and lining a loaf pan with parchment paper.
2. Next, add all the ingredients to a high-speed blender, and blend to combine.
3. Pour the mixture into the lined pan, and bake for 40 minutes or until a knife inserted into the center comes out clean.

# Spiced Cookies

**Prep Time:** 10 minutes
**Cooking Time:** 20 minutes
**Serves: 24**

## Ingredients:

2 cups of homemade almond flour
1 cup of cooked and mashed butternut squash
1 Tbsp. homemade ghee
1 Tbsp. raw honey
1 tsp. ground cinnamon
½ tsp. ground nutmeg

## Directions:

1. Start by preheating the oven to 300°F, and lining a large cookie sheet with parchment paper.
2. Next, add all the ingredients to a high-speed blender, and blend to combine.
3. Form into 24 small rounds, and place onto the baking sheet.
4. Bake for 17–20 minutes or until the edges begin to brown.

# Ginger Carrot Juice

**Prep Time:** 5 minutes
**Cooking Time:** 0 minutes
**Serves: 1**

## Ingredients:

6 organic carrots, washed
4 organic lettuce leaves, washed
¼ inch of fresh organic ginger

## Directions:

1. Simply run all of the ingredients through a juicer.
2. Enjoy right away.

**Serving note:** When first starting to introduce juice, only start with a few tablespoons, and then work your way up to a full cup only after trying the carrot juice first.

# Soothing Cabbage Juice

**Prep Time:** 5 minutes
**Cooking Time:** 0 minutes
**Serves:** 1

## Ingredients:

½ head of green organic cabbage, washed
3 stalks of celery
¼ inch of fresh organic ginger

## Directions:

1. Simply run all of the ingredients through a juicer.
2. Enjoy right away.

**Serving note:** When first starting to introduce juice, only start with a few tablespoons, and then work your way up to a full cup only after trying the carrot juice first.

# Vegetable Sloppy Joe

**Prep Time:** 10 minutes
**Cooking Time:** 20 minutes
**Serves: 4**

## Ingredients:

1 lb. of grass-fed pasture-raised ground beef

1 onion, chopped

3 cloves of garlic, chopped

3 tomatoes, chopped

½ cup GAPS homemade beef stock

1 tsp. Celtic sea salt

1 Tbsp. homemade ghee for cooking

Cooked kale for serving

## Directions:

1. Start by heating a large skillet over medium heat with the homemade ghee.
2. Add the ground beef to the pan, and sauté until brown. This should take about 5–7 minutes.
3. Next, add the beef stock, onion, garlic, tomatoes, and salt.
4. Bring to a simmer, and cook for 10–15 minutes until the stock has cooked down.
5. Enjoy with a side of sautéed kale.

# Roasted Cauliflower

**Prep Time:** 10 minutes
**Cooking Time:** 40 minutes
**Serves:** 4

## Ingredients:

1 head of organic cauliflower
1 Tbsp. cold pressed olive oil
1 tsp. Celtic sea salt

## Directions:

1. Start by preheating the oven to 375°F, and lining a baking sheet with parchment paper.
2. Next, cut the cauliflower into florets, and add to the baking sheet.
3. Drizzle with the olive oil and season with salt.
4. Roast for 35–40 minutes, tossing every ten minutes until tender.
5. Serve with a homemade soup if desired.

# Tuna Salad

**Prep Time:** 10 minutes
**Cooking Time:** 0 minutes
**Serves: 1**

## Ingredients:

½ can wild caught tuna fish in water
1 Tbsp. homemade mayonnaise
1 tsp. fresh dill
1 tsp. Celtic sea salt
Lettuce leaves for serving

## Directions:

1. Drain the tuna, and add to a mixing bowl with the mayonnaise, fresh dill, and salt, and stir to combine.
2. Serve with fresh lettuce leaves if desired, or enjoy on its own.

# Homemade Mayonnaise

**Prep Time:** 10 minutes
**Cooking Time:** 0 minutes
**Makes: About 1 cup**

## Ingredients:

- 1 cup of organic cold-pressed olive oil
- 1 organic pasture-raised egg
- ¼ tsp. pure mustard powder
- 1 Tbsp. freshly squeezed lemon juice
- 1 tsp. Celtic sea salt

## Directions:

1. Start by adding all of the ingredients minus the olive oil to a food processor or high-speed blender and blend until smooth.
2. Slowly add the olive oil, and continue to blend until the mixture thickens.
3. Store in mason jars in the fridge.

# STAGE 5

# Pineapple & Mango Juice

**Prep Time:** 10 minutes
**Cooking Time:** 0 minutes
**Serves: 1**

## Ingredients:

1 mango, peeled, pit removed, and chopped
1 ½ cups of freshly chopped pineapple
½ lemon

## Directions:

1. Simply run all of the ingredients through the juicer.
2. Enjoy right away.

# Salmon Cakes

**Prep Time:** 10 minutes
**Cooking Time:** 0 minutes
**Serves:** 10

## Ingredients:

1 large can of wild-caught salmon
1 cup of homemade almond flour (see recipe in Stage 4)
2 organic pasture-raised eggs, lightly beaten
1 stalk of celery, chopped
1 clove of garlic, chopped
2 Tbsp. homemade mayonnaise (see recipe in Stage 4)
3 Tbsp. freshly squeezed lemon juice
1 tsp. Celtic sea salt
1 Tbsp. homemade ghee for cooking
Roasted cauliflower for serving

## Directions:

1. Start by draining the salmon from the can, and add to a large mixing bowl with all of the ingredients minus the ghee. Stir to combine.
2. Form into small patties, and set aside.
3. Next, heat a large skillet over medium heat with the ghee.
4. Add the patties to the pan, and cook for about 5 minutes each side until brown. Alternatively, you can bake them in the oven.
5. Serve with a side of roasted cauliflower if desired.

# Slow Cooker Applesauce

**Prep Time:** 15 minutes
**Cooking Time:** 4 hours
**Makes: About 8 cups**

## Ingredients:

16 apples, peeled, and cored, and cut into cubes
½ cup of filtered water
2 Tbsp. raw honey
1 tsp. ground cinnamon
1 tsp. ground nutmeg
¼ tsp. grated fresh ginger
3 Tbsp. freshly squeezed lemon juice

## Directions:

1. Simply add all of the ingredients into a slow cooker, and cook on high for 4 hours.
2. Once cooked, use a potato masher to mash the apples. (This should be very easy as the apples will fall apart after cooked.)
3. Store in mason jars, and place in the refrigerator.

# Taco Salad

**Prep Time:** 10 minutes
**Cooking Time:** 15 minutes
**Serves:** 8

## Ingredients:

2 pounds of organic grass-fed beef
1 small onion, chopped
1 tsp. cayenne pepper
1 avocado, cubed
1 plum tomato, chopped
1 tsp. Celtic sea salt
Homemade yogurt for serving (optional)
1 Tbsp. coconut oil for cooking
Lettuce leaves for serving

## Directions:

1. Start by heating a large skillet over medium heat with the coconut oil. Sauté beef until brown. This should take 7–10 minutes.
2. Add the chopped onion, tomatoes, and salt. Sauté for another 5 minutes.
3. Serve with fresh lettuce leaves and the cubed avocado.
4. Top with homemade yogurt if desired.

# Tomato Soup

**Prep Time:** 10 minutes
**Cooking Time:** 30 minutes
**Serves:** 8

## Ingredients:

6 organic tomatoes, cubed
1 eggplant, diced
4 cloves of garlic, chopped
1 onion, chopped
1 tsp. fresh thyme, chopped
6 cups of homemade GAPS chicken stock
1 tsp. Celtic sea salt
1 Tbsp. homemade ghee

## Directions:

1. Start by heating a large stock pot over medium heat with the ghee. Add the diced eggplant, garlic and onion, and sauté for 5 minutes.
2. Add the remaining ingredients, and simmer for 30 minutes.
3. Using an immersion blender, blend until smooth. Alternatively, you can add the soup to a high-speed blender and blend until smooth.
4. Optional: tear up some basel to offer a slightly greener taste

# STAGE 6

# Apple & Honey Dessert

**Prep Time:** 10 minutes
**Cooking Time:** 0 minutes
**Serves: 2**

## Ingredients:

2 apples, peeled, cored and sliced
1 Tbsp. raw honey
1 tsp. cinnamon
¼ tsp. ground cloves

## Directions:

1. Start by peeling, coring and slicing the apples.
2. Drizzle with the honey, and sprinkle with the cinnamon and cloves.
3. Enjoy right away.

# Banana Muffins

**Prep Time:** 10 minutes
**Cooking Time:** 50 minutes
**Serves:** 12

## Ingredients:

2 ½ cups of homemade almond flour
¼ cup of homemade ghee, melted
3 organic pasture-raised eggs
2 very ripe bananas, mashed
2 Tbsp. raw honey
1 tsp. ground cinnamon

## Directions:

1. Start by preheating the oven to 350°F, and lining a muffin tin with liners.
2. Add all of the ingredients to a glass mixing bowl, and stir to combine, removing any clumps.
3. Pour the mixture evenly among 12 muffin cups, and bake for 45–50 minutes or until a toothpick inserted into the center comes out clean.

# Ginger Raspberry Ice Cream

**Prep Time:** 10 minutes
**Cooking Time:** 0 minutes
**Serves: 3**

## Ingredients:

2 frozen super ripe bananas
1 cup of organic frozen raspberries
¼ tsp. freshly grated ginger
1 Tbsp. full-fat coconut milk
1 Tbsp. raw honey

## Directions:

1. Place all of the ingredients into a high-speed blender or food processor, and blend until smooth. Add a splash more coconut milk if needed.
2. Split into 3 servings, and enjoy right away.

# Spiced Lamb Meatballs

**Prep Time:** 10 minutes
**Cooking Time:** 20 minutes
**Serves:** 8

## Ingredients:

2 lb. organic grass-fed ground lamb
1 tsp. allspice
1 tsp. cumin
1 tsp. Celtic sea salt
1 egg

## Directions:

1. Start by preheating the oven to 350°F, and lining a baking sheet with parchment paper.
2. Crack the egg into a bowl, and gently whisk.
3. Next, place the remaining ingredients into a large mixing bowl, and mix to combine. Add the egg, and mix again.
4. Form into 16 small meatballs, and place on the baking sheet.
5. Bake for about 20 minutes or until they are cooked through, flipping them halfway through.
6. Serve with butternut squash, or a side of roasted vegetables.

# FULL GAPS DIET

# Peach Salad

**Prep Time:** 10 minutes
**Cooking Time:** 0 minutes
**Serves: 2**

## Ingredients:

3 cups of organic arugula
¼ cup fresh raspberries
2 ripe peaches, pitted, skin removed, and sliced
2 Tbsp. chopped walnuts
4 Tbsp. cold-pressed olive oil
2 Tbsp. freshly squeezed lemon juice
¼ tsp. Celtic sea salt

## Directions:

1. Simply add all of the ingredients to a large mixing bowl, and very gently toss to combine.
2. Split into two servings, and enjoy right away.

# Avocado Egg Nest

**Prep Time:** 10 minutes
**Cooking Time:** 10 minutes
**Serves:** 1

## Ingredients:

1 organic pasture-raised egg
½ of a ripe avocado, pitted
¼ tsp. Celtic sea salt
1 tsp. cold-pressed olive oil
1 Tbsp. homemade ghee for cooking

## Directions:

1. Start by heating a medium-sized skillet over medium heat with the ghee.
2. Slice the avocado in half, and remove the pit and the skin.
3. Place the avocado in the pan, and crack the egg into the avocado. Cook until the egg begins to harden.
4. Season with salt, and enjoy.

# Apple Cinnamon Granola

**Prep Time:** 10 minutes
**Cooking Time:** 10 minutes
**Serves:** 8

## Ingredients:

¼ cup sesame seeds
½ cup of crushed walnuts
¼ cup cashews
¼ cup almonds
¼ cup macadamia nuts
2 Tbsp. chia seeds
¾ cup dried apples cut into chunks (no added sugar)
¼ cup shredded coconut (unsweetened)
½ cup melted coconut oil
¼ cup raw honey
1 tsp. ground cinnamon
1 tsp. ground nutmeg
½ tsp. Celtic sea salt

## Directions:

1. Start by preheating the oven to 300°F, and lining a baking sheet with parchment paper.
2. Add the coconut oil and raw honey to a saucepan over low heat, stir until melted, and set aside.
3. Next, add the remaining ingredients to a large mixing bowl, and stir to combine. Add the coconut oil and raw honey, and stir until the granola is well coated.
4. Place the granola on the baking sheet, and bake for 10–15 minutes or until the granola begins to brown.
5. Allow to cool before serving, and then store in mason jars.

# Chicken Sausage Patties

**Prep Time:** 10 minutes
**Cooking Time:** 10 minutes
**Serves: 4**

## Ingredients:

1 lb. of organic grass-fed ground chicken
2 organic pasture-raised eggs
1 organic apple, peeled and grated
½ tsp. onion powder
½ tsp. garlic powder
¼ tsp. freshly grated ginger
½ tsp. ground nutmeg
Homemade ghee for cooking

## Directions:

1. Combine all of the ingredients minus the ghee in a large mixing bowl.
2. Form into small patties and set aside.
3. Next, heat a large skillet over medium heat with the ghee. Add the chicken patties to the skillet and cook for about 5–7 minutes each side until brown and cooked through.
4. Serve with scrambled eggs and an avocado for breakfast.

# List of Ingredients

Organic ground chicken
Organic chicken thighs
Whole organic chicken
Pasture-raised eggs
Beef soup bones
Organic ground lamb
Organic ground beef
Wild-caught salmon
Wild-caught non-oily fish
Wild-caught tuna fish (canned)
Raw milk
Dairy kefir grains
Organic butter
Cold-pressed olive oil
Coconut oil
Yogurt starter culture
Apple cider vinegar
Coconut milk
Dill
Sage leaves
Dried basil
Fresh thyme
Oregano
Cloves
Allspice
Cinnamon
Nutmeg
Mustard powder
Onion powder
Garlic powder
Cumin
Cayenne pepper
Fresh ginger
Chamomile flowers
Parsley
Cilantro

Mint
Celtic sea salt
Shredded coconut
Dried apples
Raw honey
Sesame seeds
Chia seeds
Almonds
Cashews
Hazelnuts
Macadamia nuts
Walnuts
Mushrooms
Avocado
Arugula
Celery
Garlic
Onion
Cauliflower
Broccoli
Kale
Lettuce
Cabbage
Carrots
Butternut squash
Eggplant
Tomatoes
Spaghetti squash
Zucchini
Organic apples
Bananas
Mangos
Pineapple
Peaches
Lemons
Raspberries

# Conversion Table

## Spoon, Cups, Liquid- ml

| | |
|---|---|
| ¼ tsp. | 1.25 ml |
| 1/2 tsp. | 2.5 ml |
| 1 tsp. | 5 ml |
| 1 Tbsp. | 15 ml |
| ¼ cup | 60 ml |
| 1/3 cup | 80 ml |
| ½ cup | 125 ml |
| 1 cup | 250 ml |

## Dry Measurements

| | |
|---|---|
| 1 Tbsp. | ½ ounce |
| 1/4 cup | 2 ounces |
| 1/3 cup | 2.6 ounces |
| ½ cup | 4 ounces |
| ¾ cup | 6 ounces |
| 1 cup | 8 ounces |
| 2 cups | 16 ounces |

# Volume Liquid

| | | |
|---|---|---|
| **2 Tbsp.** | 1 fl. oz. | 30 ml |
| **1/4 cup** | 2 fl. oz. | 60 ml |
| **½ cup** | 4 fl. oz. | 125 ml |
| **1 cup** | 8 fl. oz. | 250 ml |
| **1 ½ cups** | 12 fl. oz. | 375 ml |
| **2 cups/1 pint** | 16 fl. oz. | 500 ml |
| **4 cups/1 quart** | 32 fl. oz. | 1000 ml/ 1 liter |

Made in the USA
Lexington, KY
04 November 2017